75 Day Soft Challenge

THIS JOURNAL BELONGS TO

D1710042

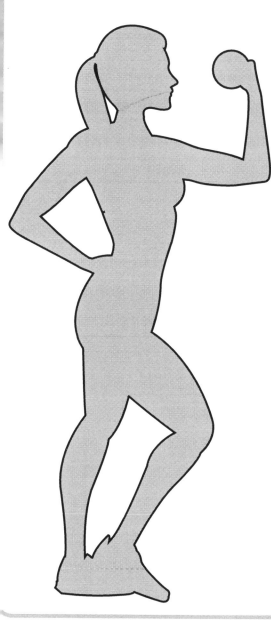

About This Challenge

the 75 soft challenge is a grogram to help ease yourself into a daily self-improvement routine .

General Rules

Eat well : Follow your plan / diet
Daily 45-Minute workout
Drink 3L water
Take a progress photo
Read 10 pages of any book

Every day do something that will inch you closer to a better tomorrow

75 Day Soft Challenge

1	2	3	4	5	6	7	8	9	10	11	12	13	14	15	16	17	18
19	20	21	22	23	24	25	26	27	28	29	39	40	41	42	43	44	45
46	47	48	49	50	51	52	53	54	55	56	57	58	59	60	61	62	63
64	65	66	67	68	69	70	71	72	73	74	75	Congratulations					

Start : / /

Weight	BMI	Arm	Waist
Hip	Thigh	Calf	Clothing size

Finish : /   /

Weight	BMI	Arm	Waist
Hip	Thigh	Calf	Clothing size

Notes :

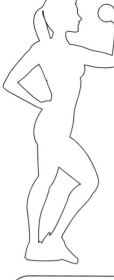

75 Day Soft Challenge

Weekly Measuruments

Week 1

	Start	Finish
DATE		
GOAL		

Weight	BMI	Arm	Waist
Hip	Thigh	Calf	Clothing size

Notes :

Week 1

Weekly meal planning

	Breakfast	Snacks	Lunch	Dinner
Monday				
Tuesday				
Wendnesday				
Thursday				
Friday				
Saturday				
Sunday				

Grocery shopping list

Notes

Day 1   M T W T F S S

75 Day Soft Challenge

- 🍎 Eat well : Follow your plan / diet   ◯ ◯ ◯ ◯ ◯ ◯ ◯
- 🏃 Daily 45-Minute workout   ◯ ◯ ◯ ◯ ◯ ◯ ◯
- 🍾 Drink 3L water   ◯ ◯ ◯ ◯ ◯ ◯ ◯
- 📷 Take a progress photo   ◯ ◯ ◯ ◯ ◯ ◯ ◯
- 📖 Read 10 pages of any book   ◯ ◯ ◯ ◯ ◯ ◯ ◯
- 🍔 Only one cheat meal   ◯ ◯ ◯ ◯ ◯ ◯ ◯

Diet Strategy

Breakfast

Lunch

Snacks

Dinner

Workout Plan

🚶 Workouts

🏃 Workouts

Reflection of the day

Physical Health	Mental Health	One way to make tomorrow better

Daily Reading

Book Title	Author	Pages
		# /

Day 2

M	T	W	T	F	S	S

75 Day Soft Challenge

- Eat well : Follow your plan / diet
- Daily 45-Minute workout
- Drink 3L water
- Take a progress photo
- Read 10 pages of any book
- Only one cheat meal

Diet Strategy

Breakfast

Lunch

Snacks

Dinner

Workout Plan

Workouts

Workouts

Reflection of the day

Physical Health	Mental Health	One way to make tomorrow better

Daily Reading

Book Title	Author	Pages
		# _____ / _____

Day 3   M T W T F S S

75 Day Soft Challenge

🍎 Eat well : Follow your plan / diet

🏃 Daily 45-Minute workout

🍶 Drink 3L water

📷 Take a progress photo

📖 Read 10 pages of any book

🍔 Only one cheat meal

Diet Strategy

Breakfast

Lunch

Snacks

Dinner

Workout Plan

🏃 Workouts

🏃 Workouts

Reflection of the day

Physical Health	Mental Health	One way to make tomorrow better

Daily Reading

Book Title	Author	Pages
		# ____ / ____

Day 4
M T W T F S S

75 Day Soft Challenge

- Eat well : Follow your plan / diet
- Daily 45-Minute workout
- Drink 3L water
- Take a progress photo
- Read 10 pages of any book
- Only one cheat meal

Diet Strategy

Breakfast

Lunch

Snacks

Dinner

Workout Plan

Workouts

Workouts

Reflection of the day

Physical Health	Mental Health	One way to make tomorrow better

Daily Reading

Book Title	Author	Pages
		# /

Day 5   M T W T F S S

Eat well : Follow your plan / diet

Daily 45-Minute workout

Drink 3L water

Take a progress photo

Read 10 pages of any book

Only one cheat meal

Diet Strategy

Breakfast

Lunch

Snacks

Dinner

Workout Plan

Workouts

Workouts

Reflection of the day

Physical Health	Mental Health	One way to make tomorrow better

Daily Reading

Book Title	Author	Pages
		# ____ / ____

75 Day Soft Challenge

- 🍎 Eat well : Follow your plan / diet
- 🚶 Daily 45-Minute workout
- 🍶 Drink 3L water
- 📷 Take a progress photo
- 📖 Read 10 pages of any book
- 🍔 Only one cheat meal

Diet Strategy

Breakfast

Lunch

Snacks

Dinner

Workout Plan

🏃 Workouts

🏃 Workouts

Reflection of the day

Physical Health	Mental Health	One way to make tomorrow better

Daily Reading

Book Title	Author	Pages
		# /

Day 7   M T W T F S S

🍎	Eat well : Follow your plan / diet
🏃	Daily 45-Minute workout
🍶	Drink 3L water
📷	Take a progress photo
📖	Read 10 pages of any book
🍔	Only one cheat meal

75 Day Soft Challenge

Diet Strategy

Breakfast

Lunch

Snacks

Dinner

Workout Plan

🚶 **Workouts**

🏃 **Workouts**

Reflection of the day

Physical Health	Mental Health	One way to make tomorrow better

Daily Reading

Book Title	Author	Pages
		# _____ / _____

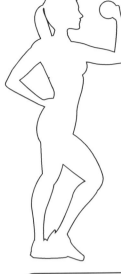

75 Day Soft Challenge

Weekly Measuruments

Week 2

	Start	Finish
DATE		
GOAL		

Weight	BMI	Arm	Waist
Hip	Thigh	Calf	Clothing size

Notes :

Weekly meal planning

	Breakfast	Snacks	Lunch	Dinner
Monday				
Tuesday				
Wendnesday				
Thursday				
Friday				
Saturday				
Sunday				

Grocery shopping list

○ _____ ○ _____ ○ _____ ○ _____ ○ _____
○ _____ ○ _____ ○ _____ ○ _____ ○ _____
○ _____ ○ _____ ○ _____ ○ _____ ○ _____
○ _____ ○ _____ ○ _____ ○ _____ ○ _____
○ _____ ○ _____ ○ _____ ○ _____ ○ _____
○ _____ ○ _____ ○ _____ ○ _____ ○ _____
○ _____ ○ _____ ○ _____ ○ _____ ○ _____
○ _____ ○ _____ ○ _____ ○ _____ ○ _____
○ _____ ○ _____ ○ _____ ○ _____ ○ _____
○ _____ ○ _____ ○ _____ ○ _____ ○ _____
○ _____ ○ _____ ○ _____ ○ _____ ○ _____
○ _____ ○ _____ ○ _____ ○ _____ ○ _____

Notes

Day 8   M T W T F S S

75 Day Soft Challenge

- Eat well : Follow your plan / diet
- Daily 45-Minute workout
- Drink 3L water
- Take a progress photo
- Read 10 pages of any book
- Only one cheat meal

Diet Strategy

Breakfast

Lunch

Snacks

Dinner

Workout Plan

Workouts

Workouts

Reflection of the day

Physical Health	Mental Health	One way to make tomorrow better

Daily Reading

Book Title	Author	Pages
		# ____ / ____

Day 9

M T W T F S S

Eat well : Follow your plan / diet

Daily 45-Minute workout

Drink 3L water

Take a progress photo

Read 10 pages of any book

Only one cheat meal

75 Day Soft Challenge

Diet Strategy

Breakfast

Lunch

Snacks

Dinner

Workout Plan

Workouts

Workouts

Reflection of the day

Physical Health	Mental Health	One way to make tomorrow better

Daily Reading

Book Title	Author	Pages
		# /

Day 10   M T W T F S S

75 Day Soft Challenge

- Eat well : Follow your plan / diet
- Daily 45-Minute workout
- Drink 3L water
- Take a progress photo
- Read 10 pages of any book
- Only one cheat meal

Diet Strategy

Breakfast

Lunch

Snacks

Dinner

Workout Plan

🏃 **Workouts**

🏃 **Workouts**

Reflection of the day

Physical Health	Mental Health	One way to make tomorrow better

Daily Reading

Book Title	Author	Pages
		# /

Day 11   M T W T F S S

Eat well : Follow your plan / diet

Daily 45-Minute workout

Drink 3L water

Take a progress photo

Read 10 pages of any book

Only one cheat meal

Diet Strategy

Breakfast

Lunch

Snacks

Dinner

Workout Plan

🚶 Workouts

🚶 Workouts

Reflection of the day

Physical Health	Mental Health	One way to make tomorrow better

Daily Reading

Book Title	Author	Pages
		# /

Day 12 M T W T F S S

75 Day Soft Challenge

- Eat well : Follow your plan / diet
- Daily 45-Minute workout
- Drink 3L water
- Take a progress photo
- Read 10 pages of any book
- Only one cheat meal

Diet Strategy

Breakfast

Lunch

Snacks

Dinner

Workout Plan

Workouts

Workouts

Reflection of the day

Physical Health	Mental Health	One way to make tomorrow better

Daily Reading

Book Title	Author	Pages
		# /

Day 13

M T W T F S S

75 Day Soft Challenge

- 🍎 Eat well : Follow your plan / diet
- 🏃 Daily 45-Minute workout
- 🍶 Drink 3L water
- 📷 Take a progress photo
- 📖 Read 10 pages of any book
- 🍔 Only one cheat meal

Diet Strategy

Breakfast

Lunch

Snacks

Dinner

Workout Plan

🚶 Workouts

🏃 Workouts

Reflection of the day

Physical Health	Mental Health	One way to make tomorrow better

Daily Reading

Book Title	Author	Pages
		# /

Day 14   M T W T F S S

75 Day Soft Challenge

Eat well : Follow your plan / diet
Daily 45-Minute workout
Drink 3L water
Take a progress photo
Read 10 pages of any book
Only one cheat meal

Diet Strategy

Breakfast

Lunch

Snacks

Dinner

Workout Plan

🏃 **Workouts**

🏃 **Workouts**

Reflection of the day

Physical Health	Mental Health	One way to make tomorrow better

Daily Reading

Book Title	Author	Pages
		# _____ / _____

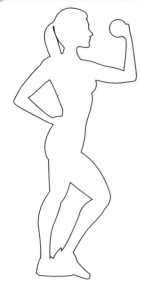

75 Day Soft Challenge

Weekly Measuruments

Week 3

	Start	Finish
DATE		
GOAL		

Weight	BMI	Arm	Waist
Hip	Thigh	Calf	Clothing size

Notes :

Week 3

Weekly meal planning

Monday
Breakfast | Snacks | Lunch | Dinner

Tuesday
Breakfast | Snacks | Lunch | Dinner

Wendnesday
Breakfast | Snacks | Lunch | Dinner

Thursday
Breakfast | Snacks | Lunch | Dinner

Friday
Breakfast | Snacks | Lunch | Dinner

Saturday
Breakfast | Snacks | Lunch | Dinner

Sunday
Breakfast | Snacks | Lunch | Dinner

Grocery shopping list

Notes

Day 15

M T W T F S S

75 Day Soft Challenge

- Eat well : Follow your plan / diet
- Daily 45-Minute workout
- Drink 3L water
- Take a progress photo
- Read 10 pages of any book
- Only one cheat meal

Diet Strategy

Breakfast

Lunch

Snacks

Dinner

Workout Plan

Workouts

Workouts

Reflection of the day

Physical Health	Mental Health	One way to make tomorrow better

Daily Reading

Book Title	Author	Pages
		# /

Day 16 M T W T F S S

75 Day Soft Challenge

- Eat well : Follow your plan / diet
- Daily 45-Minute workout
- Drink 3L water
- Take a progress photo
- Read 10 pages of any book
- Only one cheat meal

Diet Strategy

Breakfast

Lunch

Snacks

Dinner

Workout Plan

🚶 **Workouts**

🚶 **Workouts**

Reflection of the day

Physical Health	Mental Health	One way to make tomorrow better

Daily Reading

Book Title	Author	Pages
		# _____ / _____

Day 17

75 Day Soft Challenge

- Eat well : Follow your plan / diet
- Daily 45-Minute workout
- Drink 3L water
- Take a progress photo
- Read 10 pages of any book
- Only one cheat meal

Diet Strategy

Breakfast

Lunch

Snacks

Dinner

Workout Plan

Workouts

Workouts

Reflection of the day

Physical Health	Mental Health	One way to make tomorrow better

Daily Reading

Book Title	Author	Pages
		# /

Day 18

M T W T F S S

- Eat well : Follow your plan / diet
- Daily 45-Minute workout
- Drink 3L water
- Take a progress photo
- Read 10 pages of any book
- Only one cheat meal

75 Day Soft Challenge

Diet Strategy

Breakfast

Lunch

Snacks

Dinner

Workout Plan

Workouts

Workouts

Reflection of the day

Physical Health	Mental Health	One way to make tomorrow better

Daily Reading

Book Title	Author	Pages
		# /

Day 19

M T W T F S S

75 Day Soft Challenge

- Eat well : Follow your plan / diet
- Daily 45-Minute workout
- Drink 3L water
- Take a progress photo
- Read 10 pages of any book
- Only one cheat meal

Diet Strategy

Breakfast

Lunch

Snacks

Dinner

Workout Plan

Workouts

Workouts

Reflection of the day

Physical Health	Mental Health	One way to make tomorrow better

Daily Reading

Book Title	Author	Pages
		# _____ / _____

Day 20

M T W T F S S

75 Day Soft Challenge

- Eat well : Follow your plan / diet
- Daily 45-Minute workout
- Drink 3L water
- Take a progress photo
- Read 10 pages of any book
- Only one cheat meal

Diet Strategy

Breakfast

Lunch

Snacks

Dinner

Workout Plan

Workouts

Workouts

Reflection of the day

Physical Health	Mental Health	One way to make tomorrow better

Daily Reading

Book Title	Author	Pages
		# _____ / _____

Day 21   M T W T F S S

75 Day Soft Challenge

🍎 Eat well : Follow your plan / diet

🏃 Daily 45-Minute workout

🍶 Drink 3L water

📷 Take a progress photo

📖 Read 10 pages of any book

🍔 Only one cheat meal

Diet Strategy

Breakfast

Lunch

Snacks

Dinner

Workout Plan

🚶 Workouts

🏃 Workouts

Reflection of the day

Physical Health	Mental Health	One way to make tomorrow better

Daily Reading

Book Title	Author	Pages
		# /

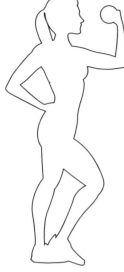

75 Day Soft Challenge

Weekly Measuruments

Week 4

	Start	Finish
DATE		
GOAL		

Weight	BMI	Arm	Waist
Hip	Thigh	Calf	Clothing size

Notes :

Week 4

Weekly meal planning

Monday
Breakfast	Snacks	Lunch	Dinner

Tuesday
Breakfast	Snacks	Lunch	Dinner

Wendnesday
Breakfast	Snacks	Lunch	Dinner

Thursday
Breakfast	Snacks	Lunch	Dinner

Friday
Breakfast	Snacks	Lunch	Dinner

Saturday
Breakfast	Snacks	Lunch	Dinner

Sunday
Breakfast	Snacks	Lunch	Dinner

Grocery shopping list

Notes

Day 22   M T W T F S S

75 Day Soft Challenge

- Eat well : Follow your plan / diet
- Daily 45-Minute workout
- Drink 3L water
- Take a progress photo
- Read 10 pages of any book
- Only one cheat meal

Diet Strategy

Breakfast

Lunch

Snacks

Dinner

Workout Plan

Workouts

Workouts

Reflection of the day

Physical Health	Mental Health	One way to make tomorrow better

Daily Reading

Book Title	Author	Pages
		# /

Day 23

M T W T F S S

75 Day Soft Challenge

- Eat well : Follow your plan / diet
- Daily 45-Minute workout
- Drink 3L water
- Take a progress photo
- Read 10 pages of any book
- Only one cheat meal

Diet Strategy

Breakfast

Lunch

Snacks

Dinner

Workout Plan

🚶 **Workouts**

🏃 **Workouts**

Reflection of the day

Physical Health	Mental Health	One way to make tomorrow better

Daily Reading

Book Title	Author	Pages
		# _____ / _____

Day 24

M T W T F S S

75 Day Soft Challenge

- Eat well : Follow your plan / diet
- Daily 45-Minute workout
- Drink 3L water
- Take a progress photo
- Read 10 pages of any book
- Only one cheat meal

Diet Strategy

Breakfast

Lunch

Snacks

Dinner

Workout Plan

Workouts

Workouts

Reflection of the day

Physical Health	Mental Health	One way to make tomorrow better

Daily Reading

Book Title	Author	Pages
		# /

Day 25

M T W T F S S

75 Day Soft Challenge

- Eat well : Follow your plan / diet
- Daily 45-Minute workout
- Drink 3L water
- Take a progress photo
- Read 10 pages of any book
- Only one cheat meal

Diet Strategy

Breakfast

Lunch

Snacks

Dinner

Workout Plan

Workouts

Workouts

Reflection of the day

Physical Health	Mental Health	One way to make tomorrow better

Daily Reading

Book Title	Author	Pages
		# _____ / _____

Day 26

M T W T F S S

- Eat well : Follow your plan / diet
- Daily 45-Minute workout
- Drink 3L water
- Take a progress photo
- Read 10 pages of any book
- Only one cheat meal

75 Day Soft Challenge

Diet Strategy

Breakfast

Lunch

Snacks

Dinner

Workout Plan

Workouts

Workouts

Reflection of the day

Physical Health	Mental Health	One way to make tomorrow better

Daily Reading

Book Title	Author	Pages
		# /

Day 27

M T W T F S S

Eat well : Follow your plan / diet	◯ ◯ ◯ ◯ ◯ ◯ ◯
Daily 45-Minute workout	◯ ◯ ◯ ◯ ◯ ◯ ◯
Drink 3L water	◯ ◯ ◯ ◯ ◯ ◯ ◯
Take a progress photo	◯ ◯ ◯ ◯ ◯ ◯ ◯
Read 10 pages of any book	◯ ◯ ◯ ◯ ◯ ◯ ◯
Only one cheat meal	◯ ◯ ◯ ◯ ◯ ◯ ◯

75 Day Soft Challenge

Diet Strategy

Breakfast

Lunch

Snacks

Dinner

Workout Plan

Workouts

Workouts

Reflection of the day

Physical Health	Mental Health	One way to make tomorrow better

Daily Reading

Book Title	Author	Pages
		# /

Day 28

M T W T F S S

75 Day Soft Challenge

- Eat well : Follow your plan / diet
- Daily 45-Minute workout
- Drink 3L water
- Take a progress photo
- Read 10 pages of any book
- Only one cheat meal

Diet Strategy

Breakfast

Lunch

Snacks

Dinner

Workout Plan

🏃 **Workouts**

🏃 **Workouts**

Reflection of the day

Physical Health	Mental Health	One way to make tomorrow better

Daily Reading

Book Title	Author	Pages
		# ___ / ___

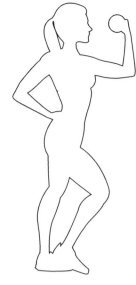

75 Day Soft Challenge

Weekly Measuruments   Week 5

	Start	Finish
DATE		
GOAL		

Weight	BMI	Arm	Waist
Hip	Thigh	Calf	Clothing size

Notes :

Week 5

Weekly meal planning

Monday
Breakfast | Snacks | Lunch | Dinner

Tuesday
Breakfast | Snacks | Lunch | Dinner

Wendnesday
Breakfast | Snacks | Lunch | Dinner

Thursday
Breakfast | Snacks | Lunch | Dinner

Friday
Breakfast | Snacks | Lunch | Dinner

Saturday
Breakfast | Snacks | Lunch | Dinner

Sunday
Breakfast | Snacks | Lunch | Dinner

Grocery shopping list

Notes

Day 29

M T W T F S S

		M	T	W	T	F	S	S
🍎	Eat well : Follow your plan / diet	○	○	○	○	○	○	○
🏃	Daily 45-Minute workout	○	○	○	○	○	○	○
🍶	Drink 3L water	○	○	○	○	○	○	○
📷	Take a progress photo	○	○	○	○	○	○	○
📖	Read 10 pages of any book	○	○	○	○	○	○	○
🍔	Only one cheat meal	○	○	○	○	○	○	○

75 Day Soft Challenge

Diet Strategy

Breakfast

Lunch

Snacks

Dinner

Workout Plan

🚶 **Workouts**

🏃 **Workouts**

Reflection of the day

Physical Health	Mental Health	One way to make tomorrow better

Daily Reading

Book Title	Author	Pages
		# _____ / _____

Day 30

M T W T F S S

	M	T	W	T	F	S	S
Eat well : Follow your plan / diet	◯	◯	◯	◯	◯	◯	◯
Daily 45-Minute workout	◯	◯	◯	◯	◯	◯	◯
Drink 3L water	◯	◯	◯	◯	◯	◯	◯
Take a progress photo	◯	◯	◯	◯	◯	◯	◯
Read 10 pages of any book	◯	◯	◯	◯	◯	◯	◯
Only one cheat meal	◯	◯	◯	◯	◯	◯	◯

75 Day Soft Challenge

Diet Strategy

Breakfast

Lunch

Snacks

Dinner

Workout Plan

Workouts

Workouts

Reflection of the day

Physical Health	Mental Health	One way to make tomorrow better

Daily Reading

Book Title	Author	Pages
		# ____ / ____

Day 31

M T W T F S S

75 Day Soft Challenge

- Eat well : Follow your plan / diet
- Daily 45-Minute workout
- Drink 3L water
- Take a progress photo
- Read 10 pages of any book
- Only one cheat meal

Diet Strategy

Breakfast

Lunch

Snacks

Dinner

Workout Plan

Workouts

Workouts

Reflection of the day

Physical Health	Mental Health	One way to make tomorrow better

Daily Reading

Book Title	Author	Pages
		# /

Day 32

M T W T F S S

75 Day Soft Challenge

- Eat well : Follow your plan / diet
- Daily 45-Minute workout
- Drink 3L water
- Take a progress photo
- Read 10 pages of any book
- Only one cheat meal

Diet Strategy

Breakfast

Lunch

Snacks

Dinner

Workout Plan

Workouts

Workouts

Reflection of the day

Physical Health	Mental Health	One way to make tomorrow better

Daily Reading

Book Title	Author	Pages
		# /

Day 33

M T W T F S S

75 Day Soft Challenge

- Eat well : Follow your plan / diet
- Daily 45-Minute workout
- Drink 3L water
- Take a progress photo
- Read 10 pages of any book
- Only one cheat meal

Diet Strategy

Breakfast

Lunch

Snacks

Dinner

Workout Plan

Workouts

Workouts

Reflection of the day

Physical Health	Mental Health	One way to make tomorrow better

Daily Reading

Book Title	Author	Pages
		# ____ / ____

Day 34

M T W T F S S

🍎	Eat well : Follow your plan / diet
🏃	Daily 45-Minute workout
🍼	Drink 3L water
📷	Take a progress photo
📖	Read 10 pages of any book
🍔	Only one cheat meal

○ ○ ○ ○ ○ ○ ○
○ ○ ○ ○ ○ ○ ○
○ ○ ○ ○ ○ ○ ○
○ ○ ○ ○ ○ ○ ○
○ ○ ○ ○ ○ ○ ○
○ ○ ○ ○ ○ ○ ○

75 Day Soft Challenge

Diet Strategy

Breakfast

Lunch

Snacks

Dinner

Workout Plan

🚶 Workouts

🚶 Workouts

Reflection of the day

Physical Health	Mental Health	One way to make tomorrow better

Daily Reading

Book Title	Author	Pages
		# /

Day 35

M T W T F S S

75 Day Soft Challenge

Eat well : Follow your plan / diet

Daily 45-Minute workout

Drink 3L water

Take a progress photo

Read 10 pages of any book

Only one cheat meal

Diet Strategy

Breakfast

Lunch

Snacks

Dinner

Workout Plan

Workouts

Workouts

Reflection of the day

Physical Health	Mental Health	One way to make tomorrow better

Daily Reading

Book Title	Author	Pages
		# /

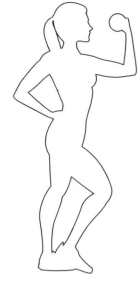

75 Day Soft Challenge

Weekly Measuruments

Week 6

	Start	Finish
DATE		
GOAL		

Weight	BMI	Arm	Waist
Hip	Thigh	Calf	Clothing size

Notes :

Weekly meal planning

	Breakfast	Snacks	Lunch	Dinner
Monday				
Tuesday				
Wendnesday				
Thursday				
Friday				
Saturday				
Sunday				

Grocery shopping list

○ _____ ○ _____ ○ _____ ○ _____ ○ _____
○ _____ ○ _____ ○ _____ ○ _____ ○ _____
○ _____ ○ _____ ○ _____ ○ _____ ○ _____
○ _____ ○ _____ ○ _____ ○ _____ ○ _____
○ _____ ○ _____ ○ _____ ○ _____ ○ _____
○ _____ ○ _____ ○ _____ ○ _____ ○ _____
○ _____ ○ _____ ○ _____ ○ _____ ○ _____
○ _____ ○ _____ ○ _____ ○ _____ ○ _____
○ _____ ○ _____ ○ _____ ○ _____ ○ _____
○ _____ ○ _____ ○ _____ ○ _____ ○ _____
○ _____ ○ _____ ○ _____ ○ _____ ○ _____
○ _____ ○ _____ ○ _____ ○ _____ ○ _____

Notes

Day 36 M T W T F S S

Eat well : Follow your plan / diet

Daily 45-Minute workout

Drink 3L water

Take a progress photo

Read 10 pages of any book

Only one cheat meal

Diet Strategy

Breakfast

Lunch

Snacks

Dinner

Workout Plan

Workouts

Workouts

Reflection of the day

Physical Health	Mental Health	One way to make tomorrow better

Daily Reading

Book Title	Author	Pages
		# /

75 Day Soft Challenge

Day 37

M T W T F S S

- Eat well : Follow your plan / diet
- Daily 45-Minute workout
- Drink 3L water
- Take a progress photo
- Read 10 pages of any book
- Only one cheat meal

Diet Strategy

Breakfast

Lunch

Snacks

Dinner

Workout Plan

🏃 **Workouts**

🏃 **Workouts**

Reflection of the day

Physical Health	Mental Health	One way to make tomorrow better

Daily Reading

Book Title	Author	Pages
		# /

75 Day Soft Challenge

Day 38

M T W T F S S

- 🍎 Eat well : Follow your plan / diet
- 🏃 Daily 45-Minute workout
- 🍶 Drink 3L water
- 📷 Take a progress photo
- 📖 Read 10 pages of any book
- 🍔 Only one cheat meal

Diet Strategy

Breakfast

Lunch

Snacks

Dinner

Workout Plan

🏃 **Workouts**

🏃 **Workouts**

Reflection of the day

Physical Health	Mental Health	One way to make tomorrow better

Daily Reading

Book Title	Author	Pages
		# /

Day 39

M T W T F S S

75 Day Soft Challenge

- Eat well : Follow your plan / diet
- Daily 45-Minute workout
- Drink 3L water
- Take a progress photo
- Read 10 pages of any book
- Only one cheat meal

Diet Strategy

Breakfast

Lunch

Snacks

Dinner

Workout Plan

Workouts

Workouts

Reflection of the day

Physical Health	Mental Health	One way to make tomorrow better

Daily Reading

Book Title	Author	Pages
		# _____ / _____

Day 40

M T W T F S S

- Eat well : Follow your plan / diet
- Daily 45-Minute workout
- Drink 3L water
- Take a progress photo
- Read 10 pages of any book
- Only one cheat meal

75 Day Soft Challenge

Diet Strategy

Breakfast

Lunch

Snacks

Dinner

Workout Plan

Workouts

Workouts

Reflection of the day

Physical Health	Mental Health	One way to make tomorrow better

Daily Reading

Book Title	Author	Pages
		# /

Day 41

M T W T F S S

75 Day Soft Challenge

- 🍎 Eat well : Follow your plan / diet
- 🏃 Daily 45-Minute workout
- 🍶 Drink 3L water
- 📷 Take a progress photo
- 📖 Read 10 pages of any book
- 🍔 Only one cheat meal

Diet Strategy

Breakfast

Lunch

Snacks

Dinner

Workout Plan

🚶 Workouts

🚶 Workouts

Reflection of the day

Physical Health	Mental Health	One way to make tomorrow better

Daily Reading

Book Title	Author	Pages
		# _____ / _____

75 Day Soft Challenge

Day 42

	M	T	W	T	F	S	S

Eat well : Follow your plan / diet

Daily 45-Minute workout

Drink 3L water

Take a progress photo

Read 10 pages of any book

Only one cheat meal

Diet Strategy

Breakfast

Lunch

Snacks

Dinner

Workout Plan

🏃 **Workouts**

🏃 **Workouts**

Reflection of the day

Physical Health	Mental Health	One way to make tomorrow better

Daily Reading

Book Title	Author	Pages
		# _____ / _____

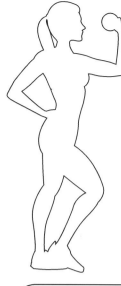

75 Day Soft Challenge

Weekly Measuruments

Week 7

	Start	Finish
DATE		
GOAL		

Weight	BMI	Arm	Waist
Hip	Thigh	Calf	Clothing size

Notes :

Week 7

	Breakfast	Snacks	Lunch	Dinner
Monday				
Tuesday				
Wendnesday				
Thursday				
Friday				
Saturday				
Sunday				

Grocery shopping list

○ _____ ○ _____ ○ _____ ○ _____ ○ _____
○ _____ ○ _____ ○ _____ ○ _____ ○ _____
○ _____ ○ _____ ○ _____ ○ _____ ○ _____
○ _____ ○ _____ ○ _____ ○ _____ ○ _____
○ _____ ○ _____ ○ _____ ○ _____ ○ _____
○ _____ ○ _____ ○ _____ ○ _____ ○ _____
○ _____ ○ _____ ○ _____ ○ _____ ○ _____
○ _____ ○ _____ ○ _____ ○ _____ ○ _____
○ _____ ○ _____ ○ _____ ○ _____ ○ _____
○ _____ ○ _____ ○ _____ ○ _____ ○ _____

Notes

Day 43   M T W T F S S

75 Day Soft Challenge

- Eat well : Follow your plan / diet
- Daily 45-Minute workout
- Drink 3L water
- Take a progress photo
- Read 10 pages of any book
- Only one cheat meal

Diet Strategy

Breakfast

Lunch

Snacks

Dinner

Workout Plan

🏃 **Workouts**

🏃 **Workouts**

Reflection of the day

Physical Health	Mental Health	One way to make tomorrow better

Daily Reading

Book Title	Author	Pages
		# /

Day 44

M T W T F S S

75 Day Soft Challenge

- Eat well : Follow your plan / diet
- Daily 45-Minute workout
- Drink 3L water
- Take a progress photo
- Read 10 pages of any book
- Only one cheat meal

Diet Strategy

Breakfast

Lunch

Snacks

Dinner

Workout Plan

🏃 Workouts

🏃 Workouts

Reflection of the day

Physical Health	Mental Health	One way to make tomorrow better

Daily Reading

Book Title	Author	Pages
		# _____ / _____

Day 45

M T W T F S S

75 Day Soft Challenge

Eat well : Follow your plan / diet

Daily 45-Minute workout

Drink 3L water

Take a progress photo

Read 10 pages of any book

Only one cheat meal

Diet Strategy

Breakfast

Lunch

Snacks

Dinner

Workout Plan

Workouts

Workouts

Reflection of the day

Physical Health	Mental Health	One way to make tomorrow better

Daily Reading

Book Title	Author	Pages
		# /

Day 46

M T W T F S S

75 Day Soft Challenge

- Eat well : Follow your plan / diet
- Daily 45-Minute workout
- Drink 3L water
- Take a progress photo
- Read 10 pages of any book
- Only one cheat meal

Diet Strategy

Breakfast

Lunch

Snacks

Dinner

Workout Plan

🚶 Workouts

🚶 Workouts

Reflection of the day

Physical Health	Mental Health	One way to make tomorrow better

Daily Reading

Book Title	Author	Pages
		# _____ / _____

Day 47

M T W T F S S

75 Day Soft Challenge

- Eat well : Follow your plan / diet
- Daily 45-Minute workout
- Drink 3L water
- Take a progress photo
- Read 10 pages of any book
- Only one cheat meal

Diet Strategy

Breakfast

Lunch

Snacks

Dinner

Workout Plan

Workouts

Workouts

Reflection of the day

Physical Health	Mental Health	One way to make tomorrow better

Daily Reading

Book Title	Author	Pages
		# /

Day 48

M T W T F S S

75 Day Soft Challenge

- 🍎 Eat well : Follow your plan / diet
- 🏃 Daily 45-Minute workout
- 🍶 Drink 3L water
- 📷 Take a progress photo
- 📖 Read 10 pages of any book
- 🍔 Only one cheat meal

Diet Strategy

Breakfast

Lunch

Snacks

Dinner

Workout Plan

🚶 **Workouts**

🏃 **Workouts**

Reflection of the day

Physical Health	Mental Health	One way to make tomorrow better

Daily Reading

Book Title	Author	Pages
		# _____ / _____

75 Day Soft Challenge

Day 49

	M	T	W	T	F	S	S

Eat well : Follow your plan / diet

Daily 45-Minute workout

Drink 3L water

Take a progress photo

Read 10 pages of any book

Only one cheat meal

Diet Strategy

Breakfast

Lunch

Snacks

Dinner

Workout Plan

Workouts

Workouts

Reflection of the day

Physical Health	Mental Health	One way to make tomorrow better

Daily Reading

Book Title	Author	Pages
		#_____ / _____

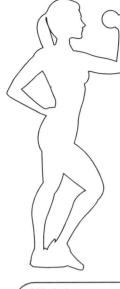

75 Day Soft Challenge

Weekly Measuruments

Week 8

	Start	Finish
DATE		
GOAL		

Weight	BMI	Arm	Waist
Hip	Thigh	Calf	Clothing size

Notes :

Week 8

Weekly meal planning

Monday
Breakfast | Snacks | Lunch | Dinner

Tuesday
Breakfast | Snacks | Lunch | Dinner

Wendnesday
Breakfast | Snacks | Lunch | Dinner

Thursday
Breakfast | Snacks | Lunch | Dinner

Friday
Breakfast | Snacks | Lunch | Dinner

Saturday
Breakfast | Snacks | Lunch | Dinner

Sunday
Breakfast | Snacks | Lunch | Dinner

Grocery shopping list

Notes

Day 50

	M	T	W	T	F	S	S
Eat well : Follow your plan / diet	◯	◯	◯	◯	◯	◯	◯
Daily 45-Minute workout	◯	◯	◯	◯	◯	◯	◯
Drink 3L water	◯	◯	◯	◯	◯	◯	◯
Take a progress photo	◯	◯	◯	◯	◯	◯	◯
Read 10 pages of any book	◯	◯	◯	◯	◯	◯	◯
Only one cheat meal	◯	◯	◯	◯	◯	◯	◯

75 Day Soft Challenge

Diet Strategy

Breakfast

Lunch

Snacks

Dinner

Workout Plan

Workouts

Workouts

Reflection of the day

Physical Health	Mental Health	One way to make tomorrow better

Daily Reading

Book Title	Author	Pages
		# /

Day 51   M T W T F S S

75 Day Soft Challenge

🍎 Eat well : Follow your plan / diet   ◯ ◯ ◯ ◯ ◯ ◯ ◯
🚶 Daily 45-Minute workout   ◯ ◯ ◯ ◯ ◯ ◯ ◯
🍼 Drink 3L water   ◯ ◯ ◯ ◯ ◯ ◯ ◯
📷 Take a progress photo   ◯ ◯ ◯ ◯ ◯ ◯ ◯
📖 Read 10 pages of any book   ◯ ◯ ◯ ◯ ◯ ◯ ◯
🍔 Only one cheat meal   ◯ ◯ ◯ ◯ ◯ ◯ ◯

Diet Strategy

Breakfast

Lunch

Snacks

Dinner

Workout Plan

🏃 Workouts

🏃 Workouts

Reflection of the day

Physical Health	Mental Health	One way to make tomorrow better

Daily Reading

Book Title	Author	Pages
		# /

Day 52

M T W T F S S

75 Day Soft Challenge

- Eat well : Follow your plan / diet
- Daily 45-Minute workout
- Drink 3L water
- Take a progress photo
- Read 10 pages of any book
- Only one cheat meal

Diet Strategy

Breakfast

Lunch

Snacks

Dinner

Workout Plan

🚶 Workouts

🚶 Workouts

Reflection of the day

Physical Health	Mental Health	One way to make tomorrow better

Daily Reading

Book Title	Author	Pages
		# _____ / _____

Day 53

M T W T F S S

75 Day Soft Challenge

Eat well : Follow your plan / diet

Daily 45-Minute workout

Drink 3L water

Take a progress photo

Read 10 pages of any book

Only one cheat meal

Diet Strategy

Breakfast

Lunch

Snacks

Dinner

Workout Plan

Workouts

Workouts

Reflection of the day

Physical Health	Mental Health	One way to make tomorrow better

Daily Reading

Book Title	Author	Pages
		# /

Day 54

M T W T F S S

75 Day Soft Challenge

- Eat well : Follow your plan / diet
- Daily 45-Minute workout
- Drink 3L water
- Take a progress photo
- Read 10 pages of any book
- Only one cheat meal

Diet Strategy

Breakfast

Lunch

Snacks

Dinner

Workout Plan

Workouts

Workouts

Reflection of the day

Physical Health	Mental Health	One way to make tomorrow better

Daily Reading

Book Title	Author	Pages
		# _____ / _____

Day 55

M T W T F S S

75 Day Soft Challenge

- Eat well : Follow your plan / diet
- Daily 45-Minute workout
- Drink 3L water
- Take a progress photo
- Read 10 pages of any book
- Only one cheat meal

Diet Strategy

Breakfast

Lunch

Snacks

Dinner

Workout Plan

Workouts

Workouts

Reflection of the day

Physical Health	Mental Health	One way to make tomorrow better

Daily Reading

Book Title	Author	Pages
		# /

Day 56

M T W T F S S

75 Day Soft Challenge

- Eat well : Follow your plan / diet
- Daily 45-Minute workout
- Drink 3L water
- Take a progress photo
- Read 10 pages of any book
- Only one cheat meal

Diet Strategy

Breakfast

Lunch

Snacks

Dinner

Workout Plan

Workouts

Workouts

Reflection of the day

Physical Health	Mental Health	One way to make tomorrow better

Daily Reading

Book Title	Author	Pages
		# /

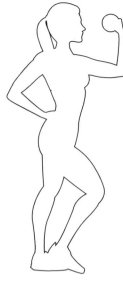

75 Day Soft Challenge

Weekly Measuruments | Week 9

	Start	Finish
DATE		
GOAL		

Weight	BMI	Arm	Waist
Hip	Thigh	Calf	Clothing size

Notes :

Week 9

Weekly meal planning

	Breakfast	Snacks	Lunch	Dinner
Monday				
Tuesday				
Wendnesday				
Thursday				
Friday				
Saturday				
Sunday				

Grocery shopping list

Notes

Day 57

M T W T F S S

75 Day Soft Challenge

- Eat well : Follow your plan / diet
- Daily 45-Minute workout
- Drink 3L water
- Take a progress photo
- Read 10 pages of any book
- Only one cheat meal

Diet Strategy

Breakfast

Lunch

Snacks

Dinner

Workout Plan

Workouts

Workouts

Reflection of the day

Physical Health	Mental Health	One way to make tomorrow better

Daily Reading

Book Title	Author	Pages
		# /

Day 58

M T W T F S S

- Eat well : Follow your plan / diet
- Daily 45-Minute workout
- Drink 3L water
- Take a progress photo
- Read 10 pages of any book
- Only one cheat meal

Diet Strategy

Breakfast

Lunch

Snacks

Dinner

Workout Plan

🚶 Workouts

🚶 Workouts

Reflection of the day

Physical Health	Mental Health	One way to make tomorrow better

Daily Reading

Book Title	Author	Pages
		# _____ / _____

Day 59

M T W T F S S

75 Day Soft Challenge

- Eat well : Follow your plan / diet
- Daily 45-Minute workout
- Drink 3L water
- Take a progress photo
- Read 10 pages of any book
- Only one cheat meal

Diet Strategy

Breakfast

Lunch

Snacks

Dinner

Workout Plan

Workouts

Workouts

Reflection of the day

Physical Health	Mental Health	One way to make tomorrow better

Daily Reading

Book Title	Author	Pages
		# /

Day 60

M T W T F S S

🍎 Eat well : Follow your plan / diet	○	○	○	○	○	○	○
🏃 Daily 45-Minute workout	○	○	○	○	○	○	○
🍶 Drink 3L water	○	○	○	○	○	○	○
📷 Take a progress photo	○	○	○	○	○	○	○
📖 Read 10 pages of any book	○	○	○	○	○	○	○
🍔 Only one cheat meal	○	○	○	○	○	○	○

75 Day Soft Challenge

Diet Strategy

Breakfast

Lunch

Snacks

Dinner

Workout Plan

🚶 **Workouts**

🏃 **Workouts**

Reflection of the day

Physical Health	Mental Health	One way to make tomorrow better

Daily Reading

Book Title	Author	Pages
		# _____ / _____

Day 61

M T W T F S S

75 Day Soft Challenge

- Eat well : Follow your plan / diet
- Daily 45-Minute workout
- Drink 3L water
- Take a progress photo
- Read 10 pages of any book
- Only one cheat meal

Diet Strategy

Breakfast

Lunch

Snacks

Dinner

Workout Plan

Workouts

Workouts

Reflection of the day

Physical Health	Mental Health	One way to make tomorrow better

Daily Reading

Book Title	Author	Pages
		# /

Day 62

M T W T F S S

Eat well : Follow your plan / diet

Daily 45-Minute workout

Drink 3L water

Take a progress photo

Read 10 pages of any book

Only one cheat meal

75 Day Soft Challenge

Diet Strategy

Breakfast

Lunch

Snacks

Dinner

Workout Plan

Workouts

Workouts

Reflection of the day

Physical Health	Mental Health	One way to make tomorrow better

Daily Reading

Book Title	Author	Pages
		# _____ / _____

Day 63

75 Day Soft Challenge

- Eat well : Follow your plan / diet
- Daily 45-Minute workout
- Drink 3L water
- Take a progress photo
- Read 10 pages of any book
- Only one cheat meal

Diet Strategy

Breakfast

Lunch

Snacks

Dinner

Workout Plan

Workouts

Workouts

Reflection of the day

Physical Health	Mental Health	One way to make tomorrow better

Daily Reading

Book Title	Author	Pages
		# /

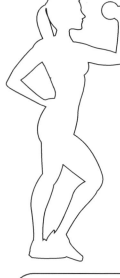

75 Day Soft Challenge

Weekly Measuruments

Week 10

	Start	Finish
DATE		
GOAL		

Weight	BMI	Arm	Waist
Hip	Thigh	Calf	Clothing size

Notes :

Week 10

Weekly meal planning

	Breakfast	Snacks	Lunch	Dinner
Monday				
Tuesday				
Wendnesday				
Thursday				
Friday				
Saturday				
Sunday				

Grocery shopping list

Notes

Day 64

M T W T F S S

75 Day Soft Challenge

- Eat well : Follow your plan / diet
- Daily 45-Minute workout
- Drink 3L water
- Take a progress photo
- Read 10 pages of any book
- Only one cheat meal

Diet Strategy

Breakfast

Lunch

Snacks

Dinner

Workout Plan

🏃 **Workouts**

🏃 **Workouts**

Reflection of the day

Physical Health	Mental Health	One way to make tomorrow better

Daily Reading

Book Title	Author	Pages
		# _____ / _____

Day 65

M T W T F S S

75 Day Soft Challenge

Eat well : Follow your plan / diet

Daily 45-Minute workout

Drink 3L water

Take a progress photo

Read 10 pages of any book

Only one cheat meal

Diet Strategy

Breakfast

Lunch

Snacks

Dinner

Workout Plan

Workouts

Workouts

Reflection of the day

Physical Health	Mental Health	One way to make tomorrow better

Daily Reading

Book Title	Author	Pages
		# /

Day 66

M T W T F S S

75 Day Soft Challenge

Eat well : Follow your plan / diet

Daily 45-Minute workout

Drink 3L water

Take a progress photo

Read 10 pages of any book

Only one cheat meal

Diet Strategy

Breakfast

Lunch

Snacks

Dinner

Workout Plan

Workouts

Workouts

Reflection of the day

Physical Health	Mental Health	One way to make tomorrow better

Daily Reading

Book Title	Author	Pages
		# /

75 Day Soft Challenge

Day 67

	M	T	W	T	F	S	S

Eat well : Follow your plan / diet
○ ○ ○ ○ ○ ○ ○

Daily 45-Minute workout
○ ○ ○ ○ ○ ○ ○

Drink 3L water
○ ○ ○ ○ ○ ○ ○

Take a progress photo
○ ○ ○ ○ ○ ○ ○

Read 10 pages of any book
○ ○ ○ ○ ○ ○ ○

Only one cheat meal
○ ○ ○ ○ ○ ○ ○

Diet Strategy

Breakfast

Lunch

Snacks

Dinner

Workout Plan

Workouts

Workouts

Reflection of the day

Physical Health	Mental Health	One way to make tomorrow better

Daily Reading

Book Title	Author	Pages
		# /

75 Day Soft Challenge

Day 68

M T W T F S S

- Eat well : Follow your plan / diet
- Daily 45-Minute workout
- Drink 3L water
- Take a progress photo
- Read 10 pages of any book
- Only one cheat meal

Diet Strategy

Breakfast

Lunch

Snacks

Dinner

Workout Plan

🚶 **Workouts**

🚶 **Workouts**

Reflection of the day

Physical Health	Mental Health	One way to make tomorrow better

Daily Reading

Book Title	Author	Pages
		# ___ / ___

Day 69

M T W T F S S

75 Day Soft Challenge

- Eat well : Follow your plan / diet
- Daily 45-Minute workout
- Drink 3L water
- Take a progress photo
- Read 10 pages of any book
- Only one cheat meal

Diet Strategy

Breakfast

Lunch

Snacks

Dinner

Workout Plan

🚶 Workouts

🚶 Workouts

Reflection of the day

Physical Health	Mental Health	One way to make tomorrow better

Daily Reading

Book Title	Author	Pages
		# /

Day 70   M T W T F S S

75 Day Soft Challenge

- Eat well : Follow your plan / diet
- Daily 45-Minute workout
- Drink 3L water
- Take a progress photo
- Read 10 pages of any book
- Only one cheat meal

Diet Strategy

Breakfast

Lunch

Snacks

Dinner

Workout Plan

🏃 Workouts

🏃 Workouts

Reflection of the day

Physical Health	Mental Health	One way to make tomorrow better

Daily Reading

Book Title	Author	Pages
		# _____ / _____

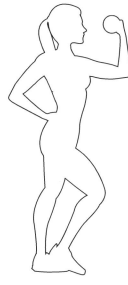

75 Day Soft Challenge

Weekly Measuruments   Week 11

	Start	Finish
DATE		
GOAL		

Weight	BMI	Arm	Waist
Hip	Thigh	Calf	Clothing size

Notes :

Week 11

Weekly meal planning

	Breakfast	Snacks	Lunch	Dinner
Monday				
Tuesday				
Wendnesday				
Thursday				
Friday				
Saturday				
Sunday				

Grocery shopping list

Notes

75 Day Soft Challenge

Day 71

	M	T	W	T	F	S	S
Eat well : Follow your plan / diet	◯	◯	◯	◯	◯	◯	◯
Daily 45-Minute workout	◯	◯	◯	◯	◯	◯	◯
Drink 3L water	◯	◯	◯	◯	◯	◯	◯
Take a progress photo	◯	◯	◯	◯	◯	◯	◯
Read 10 pages of any book	◯	◯	◯	◯	◯	◯	◯
Only one cheat meal	◯	◯	◯	◯	◯	◯	◯

Diet Strategy

Breakfast

Lunch

Snacks

Dinner

Workout Plan

Workouts

Workouts

Reflection of the day

Physical Health	Mental Health	One way to make tomorrow better

Daily Reading

Book Title	Author	Pages
		# /

Day 72

M T W T F S S

○ ○ ○ ○ ○ ○ ○

- Eat well : Follow your plan / diet
- Daily 45-Minute workout
- Drink 3L water
- Take a progress photo
- Read 10 pages of any book
- Only one cheat meal

75 Day Soft Challenge

Diet Strategy

Breakfast

Lunch

Snacks

Dinner

Workout Plan

🏃 **Workouts**

🏃 **Workouts**

Reflection of the day

Physical Health	Mental Health	One way to make tomorrow better

Daily Reading

Book Title	Author	Pages
		# /

Day 73

M T W T F S S

75 Day Soft Challenge

Eat well : Follow your plan / diet
Daily 45-Minute workout
Drink 3L water
Take a progress photo
Read 10 pages of any book
Only one cheat meal

Diet Strategy

Breakfast

Lunch

Snacks

Dinner

Workout Plan

Workouts

Workouts

Reflection of the day

Physical Health	Mental Health	One way to make tomorrow better

Daily Reading

Book Title	Author	Pages
		# /

75 Day Soft Challenge

Day 74

M T W T F S S

- 🍎 Eat well : Follow your plan / diet
- 🏃 Daily 45-Minute workout
- 🍶 Drink 3L water
- 📷 Take a progress photo
- 📖 Read 10 pages of any book
- 🍔 Only one cheat meal

Diet Strategy

Breakfast

Lunch

Snacks

Dinner

Workout Plan

🏃 **Workouts**

🏃 **Workouts**

Reflection of the day

Physical Health	Mental Health	One way to make tomorrow better

Daily Reading

Book Title	Author	Pages
		# _____ / _____

Day 75

M T W T F S S

75 Day Soft Challenge

- Eat well : Follow your plan / diet
- Daily 45-Minute workout
- Drink 3L water
- Take a progress photo
- Read 10 pages of any book
- Only one cheat meal

Diet Strategy

Breakfast

Lunch

Snacks

Dinner

Workout Plan

Workouts

Workouts

Reflection of the day

Physical Health	Mental Health	One way to make tomorrow better

Daily Reading

Book Title	Author	Pages
		# /

75 Day Soft Challenge

Congratulations

Notes :

Thank you for being our valued costomer

We will be grateful if you shared this happy experience in the online review section.
this helpes us to continue providing great products
and helps potential buyers to make a confident decision.

Our sincerst thanks

Made in the USA
Columbia, SC
23 October 2022

69888248R00057